The Unfiltered Reality of Pregnancy

An Essential Guide for Expectant Mothers

Ruth M. Smith

Table of Contents

INTRODUCTION

Chapter 1

Chapter 2

Chapter 3

Chapter 4

Chapter 5

Chapter 6

Chapter 7

Chapter 8

<u>INTRODUCTION</u>

My mum used to tell me all the time that you can never truly comprehend pregnancy till you experience it. Well after my first child I acquired a grasp of what she was saying.

Pregnancy is a unique journey—a time of deep change, growth, and anticipation. It's a period filled with excitement, dreams, and a sense of awe as a new life takes shape within you.

From the first fluttering kicks to the thrill of holding your kid for the first time, the experience is one of life's most transformational chapters.

However, amidst the well-wishes and traditional tales, there are innumerable aspects of pregnancy that often remain unwritten, hidden in the shadows of the more widely mentioned stages.

This book, "Things Nobody Tells You About Pregnancy," is designed to bring these hidden truths to light. It's a sympathetic guide that digs below the surface, examining the undiscovered waters that pregnancy can frequently steer you into. It's not only about beautiful skin and adorable baby showers; it's about appreciating the complete experience, accepting the obstacles as well as the triumphs.

Pregnancy is not a one-size-fits-all event. Every person's journey is unique, and there's no shortage of surprising twists and turns along the road. From managing the emotional rollercoaster of hormones to dealing with pregnancy symptoms that go beyond morning sickness, from the impact on your body image to the subtle intricacies of intimacy during pregnancy, this book covers it all.

We'll unearth the reality about the so-called "pregnancy glow," explore the complexities of relationships and support networks, and discuss the realities of postpartum recovery. We'll explore unexpected difficulties and address the mental health challenges that can develop, arming you with the knowledge and tools to navigate them.

Above all, this book is about empowerment. It's about giving you the insights you need to make informed decisions, enabling open conversations, and reminding you that you're not alone on this path. You'll find practical guidance, personal experiences, and a supportive network of voices that understand the intricacies of pregnancy.

As you turn the pages, you'll discover that you're not simply reading a book; you're joining a discourse that recognizes the richness and breadth of the pregnancy experience.

You'll grow to understand that the silent parts of pregnancy are just as significant as the acknowledged ones. Whether you're an expectant parent, a partner, a friend, or a family member, this book invites you to embrace the whole spectrum of pregnancy, arming you with the information and awareness to navigate the unknown with grace, resilience, and a greater feeling of connection.

Chapter 1

<u>DEMYSTIFYING PREGNANCY</u>

Pregnancy is a phase filled with wonder and anticipation, but it's also surrounded by a plethora of myths and misconceptions. Separating fact from fiction is crucial to ensure that expectant parents are well-informed and may approach their journey with confidence.

Here, we comprehensively address prevalent misunderstandings around pregnancy, offering a deeper picture of what to expect:

<u>Myth 1: "Pregnant Women Should Eat for Two":</u>

- **<u>Fact:</u>** While proper sustenance is required, the mindset of "eating for two" might contribute to excessive weight gain. Focus on balanced, nutrient-rich meals to boost your health and your baby's growth.

Myth 2: "Morning Sickness Only Happens in the Morning":

- **Fact:** Morning sickness can occur at any time of day. It's caused by hormonal swings and differs from person to person.

Myth 3: "Heartburn Means Your Baby Has Lots of Hair":

- **Fact:** Heartburn during pregnancy is caused by hormones relaxing the esophageal sphincter, enabling stomach acid to flow back. It's not related to your baby's hair growth.

Myth 4: "You Shouldn't Exercise During Pregnancy":

- **Fact:** Unless your doctor advises otherwise, moderate exercise is beneficial for both you and your baby. Engaging in safe activities enhances overall health.

Myth 5: "Pregnant Women Should Avoid All Seafood":

- **Fact:** Some seafood, specifically fish rich in omega-3 fatty acids, is excellent during pregnancy. Avoid high-mercury seafood and opt for safer ones.

Myth 6: "Sex During Pregnancy Can Harm the Baby":

- **Fact:** In a healthy pregnancy, sex is generally safe. Consult your healthcare practitioner if you have concerns or unique issues.

Myth 7: "Cocoa Butter Prevents Stretch Marks":

- **Fact:** While moisturising could assist with dry skin, genetics play a key influence in whether you acquire stretch marks. Cocoa butter can't prevent them.

Myth 8: "You Should Avoid All Caffeine":

- **Fact:** Moderate caffeine intake is generally safe throughout pregnancy. However, excessive intake should be avoided.

Myth 9: "Pregnant Women Shouldn't Dye Their Hair":

- **Fact:** Most specialists consider it safe to colour your hair during pregnancy, especially after the first trimester. Opt for ammonia-free products and well-ventilated areas.

Myth 10: "You Can Predict Your Baby's Gender by How You Carry":

- **Fact:** The technique you carry your infant is determined by your body form, muscular tone, and the baby's position. It doesn't properly predict gender.

<u>Myth 11: "All Pregnant Women Develop Gestational Diabetes":</u>

- <u>**Fact:**</u> While gestational diabetes is a risk for some, not all pregnant women have it. Regular prenatal care helps monitor and manage risk factors.

<u>Myth 12: "Pregnant Women Should Avoid All Medications":</u>

- <u>**Fact:**</u> Certain medicines are safe during pregnancy, but you should always contact your healthcare practitioner before taking any prescription.

<u>Myth 13: "Pregnant Women Shouldn't Travel":</u>

- <u>**Fact:**</u> Travel is typically safe during pregnancy, but check with your healthcare expert if you're planning a vacation, especially if it requires great distances or high altitudes.

Myth 14: "Eating Spicy Foods Induces Labor":

- **Fact:** While some believe that spicy foods can promote contractions, there's little scientific evidence to support this theory.

Myth 15: "Your Baby's Due Date is Set in Stone":

- **Fact:** Due dates are estimations based on a 40-week pregnancy. Babies often arrive within a range of weeks before or after the due date.

Myth 16: "Pregnant Women Should Avoid All Dairy Products":

- **Fact:** Dairy products are a valuable source of calcium and other nutrients. Unless you're lactose intolerant or have certain dietary limits, drinking dairy in moderation can be helpful.

<u>Myth 17: "Pregnancy Causes Tooth Loss":</u>

- **<u>Fact:</u>** Pregnancy doesn't directly cause tooth loss. However, hormonal fluctuations can contribute to gum sensitivity and a higher risk of gum disease. Good oral hygiene is crucial throughout pregnancy.

<u>Myth 18: "Pregnant Women Can't Fly in the First Trimester":</u>

- **<u>Fact:</u>** Flying throughout the first trimester is generally safe for healthy pregnancies. However, consult your healthcare practitioner and the airline's policies before going.

<u>Myth 19: "Pregnant Women Should Avoid All Hot Baths":</u>

- **<u>Fact:</u>** While too hot baths or saunas should be avoided, gentle baths are normally safe during pregnancy and can bring relaxation.

Myth 20: "Pregnancy Causes Hair Loss":

- **Fact:** Hormonal changes can influence hair growth during pregnancy, typically resulting in thicker hair. Hair loss may occur postpartum owing to hormonal imbalances.

Myth 21: "You Can't Take Antibiotics During Pregnancy":

- **Fact:** Some antibiotics are safe during pregnancy, and your healthcare expert can prescribe suitable ones if needed. Always consult them before using any drug.

Myth 22: "Pregnant Women Shouldn't Lift Anything Heavy":

- **Fact:** Moderate lifting is typically safe during pregnancy, especially if you're accustomed to the workout. However, avoid stressing your spine and employ safe lifting practices.

Myth 23: "Caesarean Births Are Less Natural Than Vaginal Births":

- **Fact:** Both vaginal and caesarean deliveries are viable childbirth methods. The choice should be based on medical factors and individual preferences.

Myth 24: "Pregnant Women Shouldn't Eat Fish":

- **Fact:** While high-mercury fish should be avoided, low-mercury alternatives like salmon and sardines are rich in omega-3 fatty acids and can be helpful for you and your kid.

Myth 25: "Pregnant Women Should Avoid All Herbal Teas":

- **Fact:** Not all herbal teas are dangerous during pregnancy. Some, like ginger and peppermint, can be calming. However, avoid teas that may promote contractions.

Myth 26: "Pregnant Women Should Avoid Exercise Completely":

- **Fact:** Regular exercise is generally safe and beneficial during pregnancy, as long as you choose appropriate activities and consult your healthcare practitioner.

Myth 27: "You Can Determine the Baby's Gender by the Shape of the Belly":

- **Fact:** The shape of the belly is controlled by various factors, including your body's shape, the baby's position, and muscle tone. It doesn't correctly predict gender.

Myth 28: "Pregnant Women Shouldn't Sleep on Their Backs":

- **Fact:** While resting on your back can potentially compress blood vessels, leading to dizziness, most experts recommend sleeping on your side to promote increased circulation.

Myth 29: "Pregnant Women Can't Have Dental X-Rays":

- **Fact:** Dental X-rays can be safe during pregnancy with sufficient shielding. However, it's advisable to postpone non-urgent X-rays until after pregnancy.

Myth 30: "Pregnant Women Shouldn't Eat Sushi":

- **Fact:** Cooked sushi and low-mercury fish substitutes can be enjoyed in moderation. Avoid high-mercury seafood and raw fish owing to potential hazards.

Dispelling myths about pregnancy encourages pregnant parents to make informed decisions, minimise unwanted concerns, and enjoy their experience with factual knowledge. By arming themselves with adequate information, parents may focus on the joy and anticipation of bringing new life into the world.

Always seek healthcare specialists for specialised advice, and remember that adopting a healthy lifestyle and keeping regular prenatal care are crucial to a joyful and fulfilling pregnant experience.

Chapter 2

<u>THE ROLLERCOASTER OF EMOTIONS</u>

If you've ever oscillated between complete, unadulterated happiness and total and utter despair, you can relate to the emotional roller coaster that is pregnancy. It's a rollercoaster voyage consisting of ecstatic highs and lugubrious lows. Buckle up — and stockpile some tissues for later.

Not every expecting woman will experience these brief moments of affective upheaval, but those soon-to-be moms who do fluctuate from rage to fear to felicity will have to learn to roll with the punches — while resisting the desire to knock anyone out along the way.

The good news for mothers struggling with ever-changing moods is: that mood swings are temporary. Eventually, you will feel like your even-tempered self again. In the meanwhile, if you want to understand why you could be blowing hot or cold at any particular moment, we have some explanations — plus a few mood-mellowing ideas.

What causes pregnancy mood swings?

There are a variety of reasons you may suffer mood swings during pregnancy — hormones, sleep loss, and nagging anxiety constitute merely the top of the iceberg.

Rest assured that you are not just being dramatic, there are real medical, physiological, and mental grounds for this seemingly unexpected activity.

Changes in hormone levels

While there are certainly several reasons leading to mood swings, the main concern is a sudden spike in irritating pregnancy hormones. During the early days of gestation, a woman experiences a veritable flood of oestrogen and progesterone. These two hormones can do a number on one's condition of mental health.

Oestrogen acts throughout your entire body and is active in the area of the brain that regulates mood - so it's no surprise that this hormone is associated with anxiety, impatience, and sorrow.

Progesterone, on the other hand, is a hormone that helps to soften your muscles and joints and avoid early contractions. Consequently, it could produce fatigue, sluggishness, and even melancholy.

So, certainly, a quick surge of oestrogen and progesterone is a recipe for the odd maternal meltdown.

<u>Fatigue and sleep deprivation</u>

First-trimester fatigue or late pregnancy sleep loss can add gasoline to the volatile fire and make it so that anything can push you off the deep end. It's hard to feel even-keeled and joyful when you're exhausted to your core.

In the first 12 weeks, "tired" is an understatement. No matter how much sleep you get, you will continue to feel depleted. This can be wearing on your body and mind — especially if you are taking care of other tiny people, performing your work, and, you know, trying to handle all those other core life commitments.

Similarly, the end of pregnancy can keep you awake at night. It's hard to find a comfortable position in bed to accommodate your swelling belly, and you are most likely suffering aches and pains or Braxton-Hicks contractions. Sprinkle on some third-trimester jitters, and it's no wonder you're tossing and turning at all hours.

Morning sickness

Morning sickness generates acute physical symptoms, but it can have major mental and psychological effects as well. It's tough to feel like your best self when you're always in fear that nausea may strike.

It's never pleasant racing to locate a restroom or empty bag to spit up in. With so many unpleasant situations — and the fear you may have to unexpectedly vomit during business meetings or whilst commuting — it can take a toll on your attitude over time.

The worry of wondering if and when your next nausea spell may hit might ruin your tranquil attitude and give way to greater stress and despair.

Physical changes

Your evolving physique could bring you tears of happiness or exasperation. Some expectant moms like watching their stomachs expand and forms evolve, others feel heartbroken watching as their bodies become unrecognisable in a matter of weeks.

The thought that a woman can develop a little person is undeniably remarkable, but everyone who has ever struggled from body image issues knows that this feat may come with its own set of challenging sentiments.

Anxiety and stress

You could be experiencing general anxiety about becoming a parent or putting another child into the mix. Stress regarding life transitions and finances could have you feeling bitter, anxious, or edgy, too.

Mounting anxiety about labour can often make a mom-to-be unpleasant or tense.

Fears about delivery are genuine and appropriate, but they can expand to become intrusive.

It's, of course, inevitable that you're going to feel a little grouchy and perpetually anxious about the misery of contractions or the future of your perineum. There are various prospective difficulties to fret about, and it can be worrisome for first-time and seasoned moms equally.

Furthermore, if you've faced troubles or loss in the past, your fear is not only normal, it's emotionally taxing. Talking to your OB as concerns arise will help to minimise some of these recurrent fears.

Are mood swings an indication of pregnancy?

If you find yourself bawling at a sappy ad one minute, and then absolutely enraged about an empty ice-cream container the next, you may be experiencing pregnancy-related mood swings — or perhaps not.

Quickly shifting emotions can be an early indicator of pregnancy. Your hormones are suddenly running, and your inability to moderate your feelings may catch you off guard. If you suspect you're pregnant, fear and anxiety can further enhance this response.

If your emotions are all over the place, and you think you might be expecting, the best thing to do is take a pregnancy test. Many women have comparable mood fluctuations before the arrival of their period, thus taking a test will give you a definitive answer one way or the other.

When will you experience pregnancy mood swings?

No two women have comparable pregnancies. While some expectant moms may suffer dramatic mood swings, others will feel emotionally stable throughout their nine-month journey. Your mood may even vary between your pregnancies.

Those who flip-flop between elation and annoyance will typically notice this emotional push and pull early on in pregnancy, when oestrogen and progesterone levels are growing, and/or late in the third trimester as labour approaches.

Many women will be excited, terrified, and eager all at once. It's little wonder your mood may vary, your life is about to change in a very major way.

What are pregnancy mood swings like?

Not all pregnant mood swings look or feel the same. You may feel bursts of joviality and times of sorrow. You could feel furious over the pettiest issue or grin uncontrollably over something absurd.

You could detest your husband or non-pregnant friends for being able to continue normal lifestyles, or you could have hidden fear over all the potential "what ifs" of labour and delivery.

If you find yourself blissfully swept up in getting ready for baby—making cribs, laundering itty-bitty onesies, and child-proofing cabinets and sharp furniture edges, your emotions may be manifesting in nesting habits. Nurture that maternal instinct and enjoy this quiet time of preparation.

Of course, it's vital to distinguish between the regular emotional ups and downs of pregnancy and prenatal depression. While there have been tremendous advancements in helping to diagnose and de-stigmatize postpartum depression, many women fail to grasp that it's also possible to feel depressed throughout pregnancy.

If you feel chronically sad, dejected, or despairing, you must talk to your doctor - for your health and that of your youngster.

What can you do for pregnancy mood swings?

Mood swings are a normal side effect of producing a mini-human within your body (and a modest price to pay), but if they're disrupting your day-to-day life at home, in the workplace, and everywhere in between, there are certain steps you can take to help you better control them.

Pregnancy is a time of significant physical and emotional development. Hormonal changes, bodily discomfort, and the expectation of motherhood can all contribute to a rollercoaster of emotions.

Coping with these emotional upheavals is a vital component of ensuring your well-being during this transforming journey. Here are extensive ideas to assist you in handling the emotional ups and downs of pregnancy:

1. <u>Self-Awareness:</u> Start by realising that emotional shifts are a natural component of pregnancy. Awareness might help you predict and manage your reactions.

2. <u>Open Communication:</u> Talk openly with your partner, friends, and family about your emotions. Sharing your feelings can give relief and establish understanding.

3. <u>Educate Yourself:</u> Learn about the hormonal changes that accompany pregnancy. Understanding the science behind your emotions can make them feel more manageable.

4. <u>Practice Mindfulness:</u> Engage in mindfulness techniques such as deep breathing, meditation, and yoga to stay present and control overwhelming emotions.

5. <u>Journaling:</u> Keep a journal to capture your ideas and emotions. Writing can provide an outlet for processing your feelings.

6. <u>Seek Support:</u> Join pregnant support groups or online forums where you can connect with others who are experiencing similar emotional changes.

7. <u>Prioritise Self-Care:</u> Engage in activities that bring you joy and relaxation, whether it's reading, taking walks, or indulging in a treasured pastime.

8. <u>Adequate Rest:</u> Ensure you're receiving adequate sleep. Fatigue can worsen emotional troubles, so emphasise restful sleep.

9. <u>Communicate with Your Healthcare Provider:</u> Discuss your emotional changes with your healthcare physician. They can

offer advice and rule out any underlying concerns.

10. <u>Partner Involvement:</u> Encourage your partner to be understanding and involved. Sharing the journey might deepen your friendship and provide emotional support.

11. <u>Embrace Flexibility:</u> Understand that your emotional environment may alter from day to day. Be flexible and gentle to yourself as you handle these transitions.

12. <u>Set Realistic Expectations:</u> Pregnancy is a season of transition, both physically and emotionally. Setting realistic expectations can help you adapt more readily.

13. <u>Engage in Creative Outlets:</u> Express your feelings through creative hobbies like art, music, or writing. Creative outlets can provide a healthy release.

14. <u>Recognize Triggers:</u> Identify situations, people, or locations that generate significant emotions. Minimise exposure to these triggers when practicable.

15. <u>Professional Support:</u> If emotional changes become overwhelming, consider talking with a therapist who specialises in pregnancy-related emotional health.

16. <u>Plan Together:</u> Include your partner in discussions about your emotional well-being. They can provide support and understanding.

17. <u>Validate Your Emotions:</u> It's okay to feel a wide range of emotions. Avoid self-judgement and instead validate your feelings as a natural part of the process.

18. <u>Stay Active:</u> Engage in regular physical activity to release endorphins, which can help regulate mood and reduce stress.

19. <u>Connect with Your Baby:</u> Create a bond with your growing baby by talking, singing, or reading to them. This connection could produce a sense of peace.

20. <u>Humor & Laughter:</u> Embrace humour and seek out activities that make you giggle. Laughter may be a strong treatment for stress.

Coping with emotional changes during pregnancy needs tolerance, self-awareness, and a proactive attitude to self-care.

By utilising these thorough strategies, you may handle the emotional swings with fortitude, generating a sense of balance and well-being throughout your pregnancy journey.

Remember that requesting support, both from loved ones and healthcare specialists, is a vital step in managing your mental well-being throughout this transitional era.

Chapter 3

ADDRESSING THE PHYSICAL CHANGES OF PREGNANCY

Pregnancy is a fascinating and altering process, both emotionally and physically. As your body promotes and supports new life, it undergoes a succession of amazing changes that are a monument to the incredible process of bringing a baby into the world.

While many elements of pregnancy are celebrated, it's crucial to have an open and honest chat about the sometimes challenging and unexpected body changes that accompany this journey.

1. Weight Gain and Body Shape:
- Weight gain is a typical component of pregnancy, crucial for the correct growth of

your kid. It's vital to know that your body is adjusting to absorb new life.
- Embrace the changes in your physical shape. Your body is doing wonderful work, and those changes are a credit to the miraculous adventure you're on.

2. Stretch Marks and Skin Changes:

- Stretch marks are a regular occurrence as your skin strains to accommodate your developing tummy. These tattoos are a testament to the strength and tenacity of your body.
- Embrace your developing skin. Use moisturisers to soothe any itching and remind yourself that these marks tell the story of your vacation.

3. Breast Changes:

- Your breasts may get larger, more sensitive, and more fragile as they prepare for breastfeeding. Your body is ready to nourish your youngster.

- Invest in comfy and supportive bras to reduce any discomfort and embrace the beauty of your body's preparation for childbirth.

4. Hormonal Fluctuations:
- Hormonal shifts can contribute to variances in your skin's look, mood swings, and even hair growth or loss. These are purely temporary adjustments.
- Remember that these hormone changes are a natural part of the pregnancy process and are a sign of your body adapting to the responsibilities of care
for a baby.

5. Swelling and Fluid Retention:
- Swelling of the feet, ankles, and hands is usual due to increased blood volume and fluid retention. Elevate your feet and wear comfortable shoes to relieve pain.
- Stay hydrated and engage in modest exercise to help minimise fluid retention and increase circulation.

6. Varicose Veins:
- Increased pressure on blood vessels can lead to the development of varicose veins. Elevating your legs and wearing compression stockings can bring relief. - Remind yourself that varicose veins are a temporary phenomenon and often improve after pregnancy.

7. Body Discomfort and Aches:
- As your baby grows, you may feel backaches, hip pain, and discomfort. Gentle pregnant yoga and stretches can help ease these discomforts.
- Embrace self-care activities like massages or warm baths to soothe your body and mind.

8. Digestive Changes:
- Hormonal changes and the enlarging uterus might cause digestive troubles like heartburn and constipation. Eating smaller meals and staying hydrated can help.

- Consider integrating fibre-rich foods into your diet to promote digestive health.

9. Fatigue and Energy Levels:

- Pregnancy requires a lot of energy from your body, resulting in fatigue. Prioritise rest and listen to your body's instructions regarding when to calm down.
- Understand that your body is working hard to nourish your kid, and rest is an essential part of that process.

10. Body Image and Self-Acceptance:

- Embrace a good body image by concentrating on the great effort your body is undertaking to nurture and grow your baby.
- Practise self-acceptance and remind yourself that these changes are fleeting and a testament to the strength of motherhood.

11. Hair and Nail Changes:

- Pregnancy hormones can cause changes in hair structure and development. Some women experience thicker, shinier hair, while others can notice hair thinning.

- Embrace these changes as part of your body's unique response to pregnancy hormones. Focus on feeding your hair and nails with a nutritious diet and delicate care.

12. Increased Blood Volume and Heart Rate:

- Your body increases blood volume to sustain both you and your baby. This can lead to a faster heart rate, especially during intensive activity.
- Listen to your body's cues and take pauses when needed. Engage in low-impact workouts that boost cardiovascular health.

13. Breathing Changes:

- As your uterus swells, it could push against your diaphragm, resulting in shortness of breath. This is a normal adaptation to fit your developing baby.

- Practise deep breathing exercises to enhance lung capacity and lessen sensations of dyspnea.

14. Dental Health:
- Pregnancy hormones could compromise your dental health, leading to
greater risk of gum disease and sensitivity.
- Prioritise oral cleanliness and regular dental check-ups to ensure dental health during your pregnancy.

15. Increased Vaginal Discharge:
- Hormonal changes can result in increased vaginal discharge. This is the body's way of ensuring a healthy environment for your growing youngster.
- Use breathable underwear and avoid douching to maintain vaginal health.

16. Changes in Libido:
- Pregnancy can lead to changes in libido due to hormonal imbalances and physical

discomfort. Communication with your partner is vital during this time.
- Keep open lines of communication with your partner and explore alternative techniques to maintain intimacy and emotional connection.

17. Braxton Hicks Contractions:

- Braxton Hicks contractions are mild, irregular contractions that can occur throughout pregnancy. They are a natural component of the body's preparation for childbirth. - Stay hydrated and modify your position if you encounter discomfort. If contractions become regular or uncomfortable, consult your healthcare practitioner.

18. Balance and Coordination Changes:

- Your changing body's centre of gravity can influence your balance and coordination. Be cautious when moving to avoid falls. - Wear comfortable and supportive shoes and consider doing prenatal exercises that increase balance.

19. Changes in Foot Size:
- The hormonal changes that relax ligaments can also produce changes in the arches of your feet, leading to a shift in shoe size.
- Opt for comfy footwear and consider using arch supports to relieve discomfort.

20. Posture Changes:
- As your baby grows, your posture may adjust to handle the increased weight. This could lead to back pain and discomfort.
- Engage in workouts that promote posture awareness and consider employing supportive pillows while sleeping.

By accepting the open discourse about the numerous bodily changes of pregnancy, you're empowering yourself with information and self-compassion. Each mutation your body suffers is a tribute to the remarkable process of creating new life.

As you negotiate these changes, remember that self-care, acceptance, and communication are your allies. Your body's modifications are a celebration of motherhood, and by honouring these changes, you're going on a road of profound transformation and growth.

Chapter 4

SEX AND PREGNANCY

If your libido is through the roof or you're never in the mood, don't be worried. An increased or decreased sex drive during pregnancy is totally normal.

Pregnancy is generally thought of as a period of fragile breasts, morning sickness, mood changes, and lethargy, but there's something more you may notice: a waxing and waning of your libido.

Rest assured, sex desire changes throughout pregnancy are natural. You may find that there are times when you can't keep your hands off your spouse (or yourself), yet at other phases of your pregnancy, sex hardly registers on your to-do list or you're put off by the thought.

But more usually than not, you'll find that your desire ebbs and flows during your pregnancy.

What causes libido changes during pregnancy?

Blame your hormones. Fluctuating levels of oestrogen and progesterone can contribute to fluctuations in sexual desire. But sickness, weariness, worry, and weight gain also decrease your libido.

(It's impossible to feel sexy, for example, if you're spending your days with your head in the toilet.) The good news is, that most women do face moments where they're more than eager to slip between the sheets with their spouses.

Increased sex urge during pregnancy

If your libido is expanding along with your tummy, enjoy your sexy urges! That rise in libido can have some health benefits for you and your baby because pregnant sex and orgasm can speed up postpartum recovery (by tightening your pelvic floor muscles) and enhance sleep and mood (it's relaxing!).

Will my sex urge rise during pregnancy?

As frequently happens with even the most extreme pregnancy symptoms, this one ebbs and flows. Some women discover that their sex desire during pregnancy is so great at times, that they're nearly always in the mood.

Don't panic, though, if your sex drive doesn't get an apparent spike. Every pregnancy is different, and it's no reflection on you or your partner.

<u>Cramps and Contractions After Sex During Pregnancy</u>

Most women believe that their libido is most likely to be revved up during the second trimester when nausea wanes and they have a bit more energy for playing. But every woman (and pregnancy) is different. If you're lucky, the surge in your sex drive could last right up until delivery day.

Causes of increased sex drive during pregnancy

Thank those pregnant hormones! During pregnancy, your breasts are getting bigger and more sensitive. Your vulva is getting engorged from greater blood flow, which can lead to more enjoyable sex. And with all that extra sensitivity, it's no wonder your sex needs may be heated up so much, even without any urging from a second party.

When is my increased sex drive likely to end?

By the time you're closer to birth, your bigger tummy — and the weariness, aches, and discomfort that come with carrying it around — may limit your ardour in the bedroom. For other women, this symptom lasts right up until the contractions start.

Just remember that everyone is different, and that just about any condition of sexual interest and frequency throughout pregnancy counts as "normal."

When should I call the doctor concerning rising sex drive?

Sex is healthy for most moms-to-be, but it's always a good idea to have a quick talk about sex with your practitioner if only to be reassured that nothing you're doing is off-limits.

If he or she has instructed you to abstain from sex for a given cause or duration, ask for specifics, especially if your libido starts to soar. Getting the information on which forms of sex are safe for you during pregnancy can assist you to enjoy yourself without worrying about any threat to the baby.

Is there something wrong with me if my sex urge doesn't grow throughout pregnancy?

Sex during pregnancy doesn't agree with everyone, and that's normal. Whether it's your shifting body, illness, exhaustion or anxiety - dread about the baby, mood swings — you shouldn't feel awful about your lack of libido

Can too much sex be bad for me or the baby?
If your practitioner has given you the green light for sex, go for it! Embrace this time and jump (make that, climb softly) into bed.

<u>Decreased Sex Drive During Pregnancy</u>

If you're never in the mood, don't panic. This is frequent in pregnancy, with over 60 percent of women reporting a reduced sex urge at some time. Rest assured, it's temporary. You would anticipate your libido to bounce back after you give birth.

Will my sex drive reduce during pregnancy?

There's no crystal ball to foresee if something will happen to you. Some women respond to hormonal swings with a revved-up libido, while others calm down.

If you've had a hard time conceiving or are experiencing a challenging pregnancy, anxiety that any sex would hurt the baby might be a barrier to pleasant playing.

When is my sex desire likely to reduce throughout pregnancy?

Research states that you may notice it the most during the final trimester when your swollen belly makes any type of movement difficult and plans for your imminent delivery make sex the last thing on your mind. But you may also experience it during the first trimester, when sickness, tiredness, and breast discomfort can put a damper on sex.

<u>Causes of reduced sex drive during pregnancy</u>

Blame pregnancy hormones and your equally perplexing feelings. During pregnancy, you could also suffer from sensitive breasts, engorged genitals (sometimes with a change in odour and discharge), and digestive issues like bloating.

Plus, you can be self-conscious about your developing size. That's normal, however, you chat with your spouse if you don't feel attractive right now because he or she undoubtedly thinks you are radiant and gorgeous. Pregnancy also makes plenty of women weary and stressed, which is hardly a recipe for excellent sex.

About 30 percent of women worry that sex or even orgasm can harm their baby or trigger preterm birth. Share your fears with your practitioner so you may be comforted that nothing that happens in the bedroom is going to jeopardise your youngster.

How long will my lowered sex desire last?

Some women who suffer a lagging sex desire during the first trimester come back strong in the second, while others endure the proverbial headache for all nine months.

If your weak libido remains post-delivery, don't panic. Research shows it can linger for up to six months after giving birth (blame restless nights and nursing), after which it promptly rebounds. If you're still not in the mood at all after six months, check in with your practitioner, who may help you sort it out.

Can too little sex be risky for me or the baby?

Abstaining totally from sex during pregnancy is fine for you and the baby. And if your spouse is feeling rejected, there are several strategies to make him or her feel loved and cared for, even if it doesn't lead to intercourse.

Is there something wrong with me if my sex drive doesn't reduce throughout pregnancy? Take your libido off your list of things to worry about. "Normal" is whatever is happening with you and your partner.

Strategies for Maintaining Emotional and Physical Closeness During Pregnancy

Pregnancy is a transforming experience that not only impacts you but also your partner. As your body and emotions face immense changes, keeping a strong emotional and physical connection with your spouse becomes increasingly vital. Here, we address several strategies to create intimacy and connection throughout this important time of your relationship:

1. Open Communication:
- Engage in open and honest talks about your views, anxieties, and expectations. Sharing your experiences might improve your emotional bond.

2. Prioritise Quality Time:
- Dedicate intentional time for just the two of you, whether it's through date nights, walks, or even simple evenings at home.

3. Share the Journey:
- Involve your partner in prenatal appointments, ultrasounds, and birthing classes. Sharing these experiences deepens your friendship.

4. Express Gratitude:
- Express thanks for the support and care your partner provides during this time. Small expressions of thankfulness can solidify your bond.

5. Physical Affection:
- Continue physical touch, such as holding hands, hugging, and cuddling. Physical affection reinforces emotional connection.

6. Love Languages:
- Understand each other's love languages and continue expressing affection in ways that resonate with both of you.

7. Engage in Shared Activities:
- Pursue interests and activities you both enjoy, ensuring you continue enjoying each other's presence.

8. Be Empathetic:
- Acknowledge that pregnancy can bring physical discomfort and emotional stress. Be empathetic and understanding toward each other's experiences.

9. Emotional Check-Ins:
- Regularly check in with each other about how you're feeling emotionally. This creates a safe climate for sharing.

10. Supportive Roles:
- Discuss how your roles may evolve throughout pregnancy and build a framework of support that works for both of you.

11. Maintain Romance:
- Keep the flame alive with gestures like surprise notes, love letters, or planning romantic dinners at home.

12. Collaborative Decision-Making:
- Involve your partner in decisions about the pregnancy, childbirth, and parenting plans. Collaborative decisions generate a sense of teamwork.

13. Share Responsibilities:
- Collaborate on household tasks and responsibilities to decrease stress and create a supportive environment.

14. Explore Sensuality:
- Explore sensuality and intimacy through activities like massage or taking baths together.

15. Listen Actively:
- Practise active listening when your spouse discusses their thoughts and feelings. Feeling heard deepens emotional connection.

16. Anticipate Changes:
- Recognize that emotional changes are a component of pregnancy. Anticipate mood fluctuations and approach them with patience.

17. Be Patient and Understanding:
- Understand that your partner may be adjusting to their feelings about the pregnancy. Patience and understanding go a long way.

18. Share Goals and Dreams:
- Talk about your objectives and dreams for the future as a family. Sharing goals reinforces a sense of oneness.

19. Laughter and Playfulness:
- Infuse fun and humour into your relationship to maintain the connection lively and enjoyable.

20. Professional Support:
- If emotional issues become unmanageable, consider receiving treatment from a couples therapist who specialises in pregnancy-related concerns.

21. Create New Rituals:
- Establish new rituals that cater to your developing needs, such as taking evening walks, reading baby books together, or having weekly check-ins.

22. Plan Future Adventures:
- Discuss and plan future adventures and experiences you'd like to have as a family. This enhances your friendship and inspires excitement for the future.

23. Manage Stress Together:
- Practice stress management tactics together, such as deep breathing exercises, mindfulness, or gentle yoga.

24. Rediscover Intimacy:
- As your body changes, find new ways to experience physical intimacy that feel comfortable and pleasurable for both of you.

25. Nurture Emotional Connection:
- Share your objectives, fears, and dreams openly. Nurture an emotional connection through embracing vulnerability with each other.

26. Explore Parenting Philosophies:
- Discuss your parenting views and expectations, connecting your aspirations for the future to develop a sense of teamwork.

27. Seek Adventure:
- Engage in activities that produce excitement and adventure, reminding you of the joy of discovery and shared experiences.

28. Laugh Together:
- Laughter is a strong technique for developing bonds. Share jokes, watch hilarious movies, and cherish joyous times.

29. Pamper Each Other:
- Take turns pampering each other with massages, foot rubs, or relaxation rituals that boost physical and emotional well-being.

30. Express Your Needs:
- Communicate your emotional and physical needs to your spouse, creating an environment where both of you feel understood and supported.

31. Support Each Other's Self-Care:
- Encourage one other to engage in self-care activities that foster mental, emotional, and physical well-being.

32. Share Your Journey Online:
- Create a shared digital location to document your pregnancy journey, allowing both of you to contribute and remark on the experience.

33. Cook and Share Meals:
- Prepare meals together and enjoy the feeling of nourishing your bodies with delicious food.

34. Express Affection Regularly:
- Continue expressing affection through simple gestures like holding hands, forehead kisses, and honest compliments.

35. Attend Prenatal Classes Together:
- Attending prenatal classes as a team boosts your understanding of pregnancy and labour, and creates a spirit of teamwork.

36. Write Letters to Each Other:
- Write letters to each other detailing your thoughts, feelings, and aspirations. These letters can serve as a valuable memento of this period.

37. Discuss Personal Growth:

- Share your individual aspirations for personal advancement and encourage each other's road toward self-improvement.

38. Be Present Together:
- Practise being present when spending time together, putting aside distractions, and cultivating focused quality relationships.

39. Share Moments of Wonder:
- Embrace moments of awe and wonder together, whether it's watching a sunset or feeling the baby's first kicks.

40. Reaffirm Your Love:
- Take time to reinforce your affection for each other via words and actions, affirming your commitment to this shared path.

Maintaining emotional and physical connection with your spouse during pregnancy is a daily journey that needs intention, effort, and mutual understanding.

By following these detailed strategies, you're establishing a partnership that will not only grow throughout pregnancy but will also set the foundation for a healthy, compassionate, and resilient family unit.

Chapter 5

<u>UNDERSTANDING PREGNANCY GLOW</u>

You may have heard of the term pregnancy glow or been assured that you have it. While it's true that your skin can appear more luminous due to a variety of medical conditions, not every pregnant woman may experience this famed "glow".

What Causes It?

It is often believed that the pregnancy glow is formed by one's tremendous happiness during the pregnancy, or from the gender of the baby. However, several physiologic factors might create that lovely pregnancy glow that occurs owing to the changes your body is undergoing.

Hormone fluctuations, Your body releases more hormones during pregnancy including progesterone, human chorionic gonadotropin (hCG), and oestrogen which can lighten your complexion.

Sometimes, they can also make your skin look flushed, giving you that glow. Increased blood flow Your baby demands blood, and your body starts generating more blood throughout pregnancy to keep up and sustain your growing youngster.

Hence, your heart pumps more blood while your blood vessels widen to permit the increased blood volume. This might cause your complexion to have that reddish hue and give you a pregnant shine. Your skin may also look fuller and brighter as a result.

Increased oil production, The fluctuations in hormone levels and an increase in blood volume could stimulate the skin to manufacture more oil and sebum. A modest layer of oil can give your skin a brilliant shine and make it look shinier, but excessive production of oil might contribute to an acne breakout in some pregnant women.

If you have a history of acne, oily skin, or combination skin, you may be more prone to excessive oil production. Heat rashes Your body temperature will naturally increase due to the changes in your hormone levels and the increased weight you're carrying because of your kid.

You may develop hot flushes or heat rashes and sweat excessively. This could bring redness to your cheeks, which can appear as a glowing and radiant look. Worsening of pre-existing disorders If you already have skin conditions such as psoriasis, eczema, or rosacea, pregnancy may increase your symptoms.

This is because your hormone levels are changing as your blood flow is increasing. The affected skin areas may look redder due to flare-ups which might be mistaken as a pregnancy glow. Skin stretching Pregnancy causes your skin to look tauter because it is stretching to accommodate the growth of your baby. Combined with the changes in your hormone levels and increased flow of blood, skin stretching can contribute to your pregnancy glow.

How Long Does it Last?

You are more likely to experience the pregnancy glow during the second trimester when your body is undergoing the biggest amount of changes. However, there is no set date as to when you will start to notice the glow.

Often, the pregnancy glow is extremely fleeting and goes away once you have given birth. Does it Happen to Everyone? Not all women get the pregnancy glow and if you don't get it, it does not mean there's something wrong with you. Your skin may just be having a different reaction to the changes in your body.

Ultimately, the pregnancy glow goes away once you have given birth, and when your hormone levels return to normal. Some ladies experience pimples and acne thanks to the increased oil production by the skin instead of getting a pregnancy glow.

In this scenario, they can opt for gentle cleansers to minimise dryness of the skin which might stimulate even more oil production. Other women get melasma or the "pregnancy mask". This manifests as brown patches that grow on your skin due to increased melanin production during pregnancy, resulting in hyperpigmentation.

Exposure to the sun typically exacerbates these brown patches but they usually go away after giving delivery when your hormone levels adjust. Women who acquire melasma often have to be extra careful to put on sunscreen regularly to prevent hyperpigmentation from getting worse.

Pregnancy glow isn't a fantasy and there are underlying physiological causes as to why many obtain it. However, not all women receive a pregnant glow and there's nothing wrong with you if you don't experience it. Pregnancy and fluctuating hormone levels could impact people differently.

Often, pregnancy glow is due to the changes in hormone levels your body is experiencing throughout pregnancy, and the increased flow of blood. Heat rashes, increased oil production, pre-existing skin conditions, and skin stretching can also contribute to the pregnancy glow. Some women may suffer acne or the "pregnancy mask" instead depending on how pregnancy changes influence their body.

They may have to take measures to reduce these instances. If you are concerned about the changes you are experiencing throughout pregnancy, consult your O&G expert to discuss your concerns.

Celebrating Your Unique Beauty

Pregnancy is a moment of profound transformation, both in terms of the growth of new life within you and the changes your body undergoes.

Amidst the bodily upheavals and emotional rollercoaster, it's vital to find and cherish the special beauty that accompanies this remarkable journey.

Embracing your individuality and the changes that come with pregnancy may lead to a powerful sense of empowerment, self-love, and an even more profound connection with the life growing inside you.

1. Body as a Canvas of Life:
- Your body's evolution is a testament to the marvel of existence. The changes you feel

are a magnificent reflection of the process of nurturing and developing new life.

2. A Symphony of Changes:
- Pregnancy brings about changes in skin texture, hair, weight distribution, and more. Each adjustment tells a tale about your body's adaptability and strength.

3. Self-Discovery:
- Pregnancy is an opportunity to reconnect with your body and embrace self-discovery. It's an opportunity to understand and appreciate what your body is capable of achieving.

4. Uniqueness in Every Stage:
- As your body develops throughout pregnancy, each stage brings its charm. Embrace the beauty of your developing tummy, the gloss of your skin, and the enthusiasm in your eyes.

5. The Joy of Nurturing:
- The love and care you provide for your growing kid are manifested in the changes in your body. This is a tangible reflection of the amazing love you're already sharing.

6. Cultivating Self-Compassion:
- Embrace self-compassion as your body adjusts. Understand that it's normal to have days of discomfort or insecurity. Treat yourself with the kindness you'd offer a cherished friend.

7. A Time of Transformation:
- Just as nature endures seasons of change, your body's modification throughout pregnancy is a part of the natural order. Embrace the ebb and flow of this amazing voyage.

8. Celebrating Imperfections:
- The stretch marks, wrinkles, and scars are reminders of the incredible tale your body is

telling. They're proof of your strength, resilience, and the particular journey you're on.

9. Capturing Memories:
- Document your journey through photographs or writings. These keepsakes will remind you of the fantastic excursion you began upon and the beauty you emanated.

10. Inner Radiance:
- The feelings and affection you have for your newborn form a wonderful aura. Embrace this inner glow that lights up your presence and displays your distinctive appeal.

11. Confidence Booster:
- Embracing your unique appeal throughout pregnancy will enhance your self-confidence. Recognizing the strength and beauty in your body builds a healthy self-image.

12. Bonding with Your Baby:
- Embracing your unique beauty during pregnancy also bonds you to your baby. Your body is the vessel that nurtures and protects, forming an unbreakable relationship.

13. Shifting Perspectives:
- Focus on the marvel of life blossoming within you. Shifting your outlook from external appearance to the magic within can transform your self-perception.

14. Empowerment Through Acceptance:
- Accepting and enjoying your changing body enables you to focus on what is important – the health and well-being of you and your kid.

15. Setting a Positive Example:
- By embracing your unique appeal, you set a terrific example for your child. You

educate them that self-love and acceptance are vital components of a healthy mentality.

Embracing your unique beauty throughout pregnancy is not only a superficial gesture; it's a significant journey of self-discovery, self-love, and empowerment. By enjoying the beauty inside the changes, you're honouring the essence of life itself.

As you embrace your personality and the journey of pregnancy, you're constructing a legacy of love, acceptance, and empowerment for yourself and the generations to come. Remember that your unique beauty is a reflection of the magnificent journey you're travelling – one that leads to the production of new life and the flowering of an even more lovely you.

Chapter 6

<u>NAVIGATING HEALTH CHALLENGES DURING PREGNANCY</u>

Pregnancy is a changing experience filled with wonder and anticipation, but it can also come with its share of health challenges.

Understanding these potential concerns and obtaining correct care helps preserve the well-being of both you and your growing youngster. Here, we dive deeper into the different health concerns that could emerge during pregnancy, offering insights into their causes, symptoms, and management:

1. Morning Sickness with Hyperemesis Gravidarum:
- Morning sickness is frequent, with symptoms like nausea and vomiting. In severe cases, hyperemesis gravidarum can

lead to excessive vomiting, dehydration, and weight loss.

2. Gestational Diabetes:
- Hormonal changes can lead to insulin resistance, generating higher blood sugar levels. Proper control through food, exercise, and medicine can decrease dangers.

3. Preeclampsia:
- This syndrome involves excessive blood pressure and organ damage, often occurring in the latter half of pregnancy. Regular prenatal care is crucial for early detection.

4. Anaemia:
- Iron-deficiency anaemia is common during pregnancy due to increased blood volume. Supplements and iron-rich diets can help prevent and manage it.

5. Urinary Tract Infections (UTIs):
- Hormonal changes can make pregnant women more prone to UTIs. Prompt treatment is vital to avert issues.

6. Back Pain and Sciatica:
- As the body adjusts to the increasing belly, back discomfort and sciatica can arise due to strain on the nerves. Proper posture, exercises, and prenatal yoga can bring help.

7. Varicose Veins and Haemorrhoids:
- Increased blood volume and pressure can contribute to varicose veins and haemorrhoids. Elevating legs, being moving, and avoiding prolonged standing will help.

8. Constipation:
- Hormones and pressure on the digestive tract can cause constipation. A high-fibre diet, water, and mild exercises help ease this condition.

9. Heartburn and Indigestion:
- Hormonal shifts might loosen the lower esophageal sphincter, causing heartburn. Smaller, more frequent meals and avoiding trigger foods can help.

10. Stretch Marks:
- Rapid growth and straining of the skin could lead to stretch marks. While they're frequent, keeping the skin hydrated with moisturisers helps decrease their appearance.

11. Swelling and Edema:
- Fluid retention and pressure on blood vessels can cause swelling in the feet, ankles, and hands. Elevating legs and being active can help reduce swelling.

12. Sleep Disruptions:
- Hormonal changes, discomfort, and frequent restroom excursions could impair sleep. Creating a bedtime routine and

adopting supportive pillows can aid in restful sleep.

13. Shortness of Breath:
- As the uterus swells, it could press against the diaphragm, generating shortness of breath. Focus on excellent breathing strategies and prevent overexertion.

14. Mood Changes and Anxiety:
- Hormones and emotional upheavals could lead to mood swings and anxiety. Open interaction with loved ones and seeking support are vital.

15. Depression and Perinatal Mood Disorders:
- Depression during pregnancy, known as perinatal depression, is a major concern. Professional aid, counselling, and drugs can bring relief.

16. Carpal Tunnel Syndrome:
- Swelling and fluid retention can contribute to carpal tunnel syndrome. Wrist exercises and splints can minimise discomfort.

17. Leg Cramps:
- Hormonal fluctuations and pressure on nerves could trigger leg cramps. Staying hydrated and mild stretching can help prevent cramps.

18. Pelvic Girdle Pain:
- Hormonal changes and the mobility of the pelvic bones could cause discomfort. Prenatal workouts and physical therapy can bring support.

19. Insomnia:
- Hormonal swings, discomfort, and concern can lead to insomnia. Practising relaxation techniques and maintaining a consistent sleep cycle can assist.

20. Dizziness and Fainting:
- Changes in blood pressure and circulation could contribute to dizziness and fainting. Avoid standing for lengthy durations and rise slowly from sitting or reclining postures.

21. Vaginal Discomfort and Infections:
- Hormonal variations could influence vaginal pH, leading to discomfort and increased susceptibility to infections. Maintaining good hygiene and wearing breathable clothing might assist prevent issues.

22. Breast Changes and Tenderness:
- Hormones prepare the body for breastfeeding, promoting breast development and pain. Supportive bras and gentle breast massages could ease discomfort.

23. Nausea and Vomiting:
- Nausea and vomiting, widely known as morning sickness, can be hard. Eating modest, regular meals and staying hydrated can manage symptoms.

24. Joint and Ligament Pain:
- The hormone relaxin can cause joints and ligaments to soften, resulting in discomfort. Prenatal workouts and avoiding hard activities can bring relief.

25. Gum and Dental Issues:
- Hormonal fluctuations could damage gum health, creating bleeding and sensitivity. Regular dental care and adequate oral hygiene are crucial throughout pregnancy.

26. Skin Changes and Acne:
- Hormones can lead to skin changes, including acne. Using mild skincare products and following a consistent routine can help treat skin concerns.

27. High Blood Pressure:
- Developing high blood pressure during pregnancy could lead to complications like preeclampsia. Regular monitoring and attention to healthcare suggestions are crucial.

28. Allergies and Respiratory Issues:
- Pregnancy-related hormonal changes could aggravate allergies and respiratory issues. Avoiding triggers and seeking a healthcare specialist for safe treatments is crucial.

29. Thyroid Issues:
- Pregnancy can decrease thyroid function. Regular thyroid exams and adequate therapy are crucial to ensure a healthy pregnancy.

30. Incontinence:
- Hormonal changes and pressure on the bladder might cause urine incontinence.

Pelvic floor exercises and cautious water can help control this condition.

31. Abdominal Pain
- As the uterus expands, stomach discomfort is frequent. However, significant or chronic discomfort should be reported to a healthcare provider.

32. Haemorrhoids:
- Increased pressure on blood vessels could lead to haemorrhoids. Hydration, a high-fibre diet, and avoiding straining during bowel motions can prevent this condition.

33. Vaginal Bleeding:
- Light spotting can be usual throughout pregnancy, but severe or chronic bleeding requires immediate medical treatment.

34. Preterm Labour:
- Contractions and labour before 37 weeks are considered preterm. Recognizing the

indicators and seeking medical treatment immediately is crucial.

35. Placental Issues:
- Placental abruption or previa can pose issues. Regular prenatal care and early identification are crucial to handle these issues.

36. Itching and Skin Conditions:
- Hormonal shifts could promote itching and skin diseases. Consult a healthcare provider for safe solutions to tackle these challenges.

37. Vaginal Discharge:
- Changes in vaginal discharge are frequent throughout pregnancy. While modest modifications are frequent, unexpected or foul-smelling discharge should be addressed with a healthcare practitioner.

38. Vision Changes:
- Fluid retention can change eye shape and eyesight. Regular eye check-ups and limiting fluid retention can lessen visual difficulties.

39. Braxton Hicks Contractions:
- These practice contractions can be mistaken for true labour. Staying hydrated, changing positions, and relaxation can ease discomfort.

40. Fatigue:
- Hormonal changes and increased energy needs could lead to tiredness. Rest, appropriate nutrition, and regular exercise can alleviate pregnancy-related weariness.

Navigating the myriad health risks that could emerge during pregnancy involves awareness, proactive treatment, and open communication with healthcare providers. Remember that you're not alone on this road; seek help, support, and correct therapy as needed.

By prioritising your well-being and being informed, you may overcome these issues and focus on the lovely experience of bringing new life into the world. Each worry you address is a testimonial to your dedication to the health and happiness of both you and your baby.

STRATEGIES FOR COPING AND THRIVING

Pregnancy is a time of hope and enthusiasm, although unanticipated health concerns could occur, casting a shadow over this precious journey.

Coping with these difficulties requires resilience, knowledge, and a supportive network. Here, we completely discuss strategies to cope with unforeseen health concerns during pregnancy, helping you to transcend these trials with courage and grace:

1. Stay Informed and Seek Professional Help:
- Knowledge is power. Educate yourself about normal pregnancy-related illnesses and accompanying symptoms. If you encounter unexpected symptoms, consult your healthcare expert quickly. They can give credible information and advice.

2. Prioritise Open Communication:
- Talk truthfully with your healthcare practitioner about your concerns and symptoms. Clear communication ensures you receive timely and appropriate care. Share your fears with your partner, family, and friends for emotional support.

3. Practice Self-Compassion:
- Pregnancy is a unique adventure, and problems are a natural part of it. Be gentle to yourself and understand that unplanned hardships are not your fault. Embrace

self-love and remember that you're doing your best.

4. Build a Support System:
- Surround yourself with a supportive network of family, friends, and healthcare professionals. Their understanding, sympathy, and practical aid can make a huge difference in your journey.

5. Educate Yourself About Your Condition:
- Learn about the health difficulties you're facing. Understand its causes, expected effects, and possible treatment possibilities. Knowledge helps you to make intelligent decisions and actively engage in your therapy.

6. Practice Mindfulness and Stress Reduction:
- Coping with unforeseen health difficulties could produce stress and worry. Engage in mindfulness techniques, meditation, deep

breathing, and light activities to regulate tension and promote relaxation.

7. Adapt Your Lifestyle as Needed:
- If your health requires lifestyle modifications, embrace them as part of your temporary reality. Modify your cuisine, fitness routine, and everyday activities to meet your demands.

8. Maintain a Healthy Routine:
- Adhering to a balanced diet, staying hydrated, and obtaining regular exercise can add to your general well-being and assist in handling unforeseen health challenges.

9. Stay Positive and Focus on the Future:
- While it's natural to feel overwhelmed, adopt an optimistic perspective. Remind yourself that challenges are ephemeral, and your ultimate purpose is the well-being of both you and your kid.

10. Seek Professional Psychological Support:
- If you're struggling to manage emotionally, try getting the support of a therapist or counsellor. Professional support can provide strategies to manage stress and anxiety properly.

11. Lean on Online Support Communities:
- Online forums and support groups for pregnant individuals suffering health concerns can give a secure location to share tales, receive advice, and connect with others who understand.

12. Set Realistic Expectations:
- Understand that not every day will be the same. Set reasonable expectations for yourself and recognize that some days may be more tough than others.

13. Focus on the Silver Linings:
- While confronting unanticipated health challenges could be worrisome, it can also present an opportunity for personal growth,

courage, and a greater relationship with your youngster.

14. Document Your Journey:
- Keeping a journal or blog can help you manage your feelings, document your progress, and reflect on your journey's highs and lows.

15. Celebrate Small Victories:
- Every action you take to manage an unplanned health issue is a triumph. Celebrate each milestone, no matter how modest, as a tribute to your strength.

Coping with unanticipated health difficulties during pregnancy involves a combination of self-compassion, education, and support. By accepting these strategies, you're not only navigating the challenges with perseverance but also establishing a good example for your infant.

Remember that you're not alone on this road; reach out for aid, draw on your support network, and focus on the enormous strength that resides inside you.

Through solid coping skills and a determined mindset, you may manage these obstacles and emerge from them with a deeper sense of empowerment and an even tighter bond with your developing youngster.

Chapter 7

THE CONCEPT OF LABOR

Labour is the procedure during which a foetus and placenta are expelled from the uterus through the vagina.

Human labour is separated into three parts. The initial stage is further split into two components. Successful labour includes three factors: the mother's efforts and uterine contractions, foetal characteristics, and pelvic structure.

This trinity is commonly referred to as the passenger, power, and passage. Clinicians often deploy many techniques to monitor labour. Serial cervical examinations are performed to determine cervical dilation, effacement, and foetal position, often known as the station.

Foetal cardiac monitoring is performed nearly continuously to determine foetal well-being throughout delivery. Cardiotocography is used to monitor the frequency and adequacy of contractions. Medical workers use the information they collect from monitoring and cervical exams to identify the patient's stage of labour and follow labour progression.

Initial Evaluation and Presentation of Labor Women will regularly self-present to obstetrical triage with worry about the onset of labour. Common primary complaints include painful contractions, vaginal bleeding/bloody show, and fluid leaks from the vagina.

It is up to the clinician to determine if the patient is in labour, defined as regular, clinically meaningful contractions with an objective change in cervical dilatation and/or effacement.

When women are first present at the labour and delivery unit, vital signs, including temperature, heart rate, oxygen saturation, breathing rate, and blood pressure, should be taken and checked for any anomalies.

The patient should be placed on continuous cardiotocographic monitoring to guarantee foetal wellbeing. The patient's prenatal record, including obstetric history, surgical history, medical history, laboratory, and imaging data, should undergo review. Finally, a history of present illness, review of systems, and physical exam, including a sterile speculum exam, will need to take place.

During the sterile speculum exam, clinicians will check for indicators of rupture of membranes such as amniotic fluid accumulating in the posterior vaginal canal. If the doctor is unsure whether or not a rupture of membranes has occurred, additional testing such as pH testing, microscopic exam searching for ferning of the fluid, or laboratory testing of the fluid can be the next step.

Amniotic fluid has a pH of 7.0 to 7.5, which is more basic than typical vaginal pH. A sterile gloved exam should be done to establish the degree of cervical dilatation and effacement. The measurement of cervical dilation is achieved by finding the external cervical os and spreading one's fingers in a 'V' shape, then estimating the distance in centimetres between the two fingers.

Effacement is determined by calculating the percentage remaining of the length of the thinned cervix compared to the uneffaced cervix. During the cervical exam, confirmation of the presenting foetal part is also necessary.

Bedside ultrasonography can be used to confirm the presentation and position of the foetal presenting part. Particular attention should be made in the case of breech presentation due to its heightened risks of foetal morbidity and death compared with the cephalic-presenting foetus.

Management of Normal Labor

Labour is a normal process, however it might suffer interruption by complicated situations, which at times necessitate therapeutic intervention. The treatment of low-risk labour is a careful balance between letting the natural process proceed and limiting any potential difficulties.

During labour, cardiotocographic monitoring is commonly conducted to measure uterine contractions and foetal heart rate throughout time. Clinicians watch foetal heart tracings to evaluate for any symptoms of foetal discomfort that would necessitate intervention as well as the adequacy or inadequacy of contractions.

Vital signs of the mother are collected at regular intervals and whenever concerns occur regarding a clinical status change. Laboratory testing often includes the haemoglobin, hematocrit, and platelet count and is sometimes repeated following delivery if serious blood loss occurs. Cervical exams are generally performed every 2 to 3 hours unless concerns emerge and require more frequent exams.

Frequent cervical checks are related with an increased risk of infection, especially if a rupture of membranes has occurred. Women should be permitted to ambulate freely and change postures if desired.

An intravenous catheter is commonly placed in case it is required to give medications or fluids. Oral intake should not be withheld. If the patient remains without food or drink for a longer amount of time, intravenous fluids should be considered to help replenish losses but do not need to be used continually on all labouring patients.

Analgesia is administered in the form of intravenous opioids, inhaled nitrous oxide, and neuraxial analgesia in those who are appropriate candidates.

Amniotomy is considered on an as-needed basis for foetal scalp monitoring or labour augmentation, but its habitual use should be discouraged. Oxytocin may be initiated to increase contractions judged to be inadequate.

First Stage of Labor

The first stage of labour begins when labour starts and finishes with full cervical dilation to 10 centimetres. Labour often begins spontaneously or may be induced medically for a variety of maternal or foetal indications. Methods of initiating labour include cervical ripening with prostaglandins, membrane stripping, amniotomy, and intravenous oxytocin.

Although precisely defining when labour starts may be inexact, labour is generally defined as beginning when contractions become intense and regularly spaced at roughly 3 to 5 minutes apart.

Women may feel uncomfortable contractions throughout pregnancy that do not progress to cervical dilation or effacement, referred to as false labour. Thus, determining the onset of employment often relies on retrospective or subjective evidence. Friedman et al. were some of the first to examine labour progress and classified the commencement of labour as starting when women felt significant and regular contractions.

He graphed cervical dilation over time and determined that typical labour has a sigmoidal curve. Based on the information from his labour graphs, he claimed that labour has three divisions. First, a preparatory stage defined by gradual cervical dilatation, with major biochemical and structural alterations.

This is also known as the latent phase of the first stage of labour. Second, a substantially shorter and rapid dilational phase is also known as the active phase of the first stage of labour. Third, a pelvic division phase, which occurs during the second stage of labour.

The first stage of labour is further classified into two phases, distinguished by the degree of cervical dilation. The latent phase is commonly classed as 0 to 6 cm, while the active phase commences from 6 cm to full cervical dilation. The displaying foetal component also begins the process of engagement into the pelvis during the first stage.

Throughout the early stage of labour, serial cervical exams are done to identify the location of the foetus, cervical dilation, and cervical effacement. Cervical effacement refers to the cervical length in the anterior-posterior plane. When the cervix has fully thinned out, and no length is left, this is referred to as 100 percent effacement.

The station of the foetus is defined relative to its position in the maternal pelvis. When the bony foetal presenting portion is aligned with the maternal ischial spine, the foetus is 0 station. Proximal to the ischial spines are stations -1 cm to -5 centimetres, and distal to the ischial spines are +1 to +5 stations.

The first stage of labour involves a latent period and an active phase. During the latent phase, the cervix dilates gently to around 6 cm. The latent phase is generally much longer and less predictable in relation to the rate of cervical change than is observed in the active phase. A normal latent phase can continue up to 20 hours and 14 hours in nulliparous and multiparous women, respectively, without being deemed extended.

Sedation can increase the duration of the latent phase of labour. The cervix changes more rapidly and predictably in the active phase until it reaches 10 centimetres and cervical dilatation and effacement are complete. Active labour with faster cervical dilation commonly starts at 6 cm of dilation.

During the active phase, the cervix generally dilated at a pace of 1.2 to 1.5 centimetres per hour. Multiparas, or women with a history of past vaginal delivery, tend to display more fast cervical dilatation. The absence of cervical change for greater than 4 hours in the midst of adequate contractions or six hours with inadequate contractions is considered the arrest of labour and may justify clinical intervention.

Second Stage of Labor

The second stage of labour commences with complete cervical dilation to 10 cm and finishes with the delivery of the newborn. This was also defined as the pelvic division phase by Friedman. After cervical dilation is complete, the foetus descends into the vaginal canal with or without maternal pushing efforts.

The foetus passes through the birth canal via 7 movements known as the cardinal movements. These include engagement, descent, flexion, internal rotation, extension, external rotation, and expulsion. In women who have delivered vaginally previously, whose bodies have adjusted to delivering a foetus, the second stage may only take a brief trial, however a greater length may be required for a nulliparous female.

In patients without neuraxial anaesthesia, the second stage of labour often lasts less than three hours in nulliparous women and less than two hours in multiparous women. In women who get neuraxial anaesthesia, the second stage of labour generally lasts less than four hours in nulliparous women and fewer than three hours in multiparous women.

If the second stage of labour lasts longer than these criteria, then the second stage is termed protracted. Several components may influence the duration of the second stage of labour, including foetal parameters such as foetal size and position, mother factors such as pelvic shape, the number of expulsive efforts, comorbidities such as hypertension or diabetes, age, and history of previous deliveries.

Third Stage of Labor

The third stage of labour occurs after the foetus is delivered and concludes with the birth of the placenta. Separation of the placenta from the uterine interface is hallmarked by three cardinal indicators, including a gush of blood at the vagina, extension of the umbilical cord, and a globular-shaped uterine fundus on probing.

Spontaneous ejection of the placenta normally takes between 5 to 30 minutes. A delivery time of greater than 30 minutes is connected with a higher risk of postpartum haemorrhage and may be a signal for manual removal or other intervention. Management of the third stage of labour requires applying traction on the umbilical cord with concomitant fundal pressure to promote speedier placental delivery.

The purpose of the stages of labour is to establish a universal description that medical practitioners may use to communicate with one other about labour. The phases of labour can be employed to assist in assessing where the patient is on the labour spectrum. Clarifying the stages of labour has helped develop suggestions, which identify usual and aberrant trends in labour. Clinical management also caters toward the various stages of labour.

Complications may occur during any of the stages of labour to result in abnormal labour. During the first stage, women may experience the arrest of parturition, necessitating caesarean birth, which may offer a larger maternal or foetal danger. Second-stage issues include a range of complications due to the shock of the delivery process to either the foetus or the mother.

The foetus can experience acidemia, shoulder dystocia, bone fractures, nerve palsies, scalp hematomas, and anoxic brain damage. Similarly, the mother can experience a range of serious effects ranging from uterine rupture, vaginal laceration, cervical laceration, uterine haemorrhage, amniotic fluid embolism, and death. The third stage of labour may encounter complications from haemorrhage, cord avulsion, retained placenta, or incomplete evacuation of the placenta.

Defining the stages of labour with a definite beginning and finish has allowed clinicians to examine labour trends and develop labour curves. For example, in the 1950s, Dr. Friedman produced a graphical representation of the rate of normal labour during latent and active labour using observed clinical data.

These, in turn, can be used to evaluate if a woman is advancing through labour as planned and aid to diagnose atypical labour. Friedman noted that labour often had a sigmoidal curve when evaluated by cervical dilation over time. During the active phase of labour, cervical dilatation happens at a pace of 1 centimetre or more each hour. If dilation occurs substantially slowly, the patient may be at risk for atypical labour or arrest of labour.

If a woman is found not going through the initial stage of labour as predicted, this could lead to the diagnosis of the arrest of dilatation or descent, which could result in caesarean birth. The findings of Dr. Friedman have lately been questioned, and the current view is that the usual latent phase of labour lasts longer than was previously documented.

The criteria for the stages of labour generate a universal language that allows healthcare practitioners to communicate with one another regarding patient care accurately. Also, various medicines are customised to particular stages of labour to try to obtain better patient results.

For example, active management in the third stage of labour is carried out by applying rapid traction on the umbilical cord and delivering intravenous oxytocin, which correlates with a lower risk of postpartum haemorrhage. Clinicians will continue to use the stages of labour to guide labour management and investigate labour patterns to improve patient care.

Enhancing Healthcare Team Outcomes

The phases of labour represent a complex physiologic process that starts when labour begins and finishes with the delivery of the foetus and placenta. Labour is regularly monitored clinically with numerous modalities by an interprofessional team. The process of labour can continue as widely assumed with specific cardinal events and time constraints or can confront issues and delays, which may require identification and medical intervention.

The presence of the interprofessional team in monitoring and caring for women throughout labour is vital in keeping women safe and enhancing outcomes during the labour process.

A wide array of medical experts such as nurses, midwives, pharmacists, family physicians, anesthesiologists, and obstetrician/gynaecologists may be engaged in a woman's labour process. Close communication is required between these individuals to maintain an atmosphere of safety and patient-centred care.

Midwives generally supervise labour and delivery and work closely with physicians when difficulties emerge, requiring physician intervention, such as the Caesarian section or surgical delivery. Pharmacists ensure that patients acquire the correct analgesics, tocolytics, and other medications that may be needed during or following childbirth.

Anesthesiologists and nurse anaesthetists give epidurals for analgesia and are available for general endotracheal anaesthesia when necessary. Nurses monitor the patient's vital signs, contractions, cervical examinations, and pain scores, dispense medicines, notice issues, and update the physician or midwife responsible for the patient.

Each childbirth is unique, but an interprofessional approach prenatally and throughout labour can be used to improve patient outcomes and provide patient-centred care, as each provider class works collaboratively to ensure communication lines remain open between different disciplines on the health care team.

Navigating the Unpredictable: Unexpected Outcomes, Pain Management, and the Realities of Childbirth

Childbirth, a crucial event that usher's new life into the world, is a journey marked by its own set of hardships, uncertainty, and changing experiences.

While the thought of welcoming a newborn is filled with enthusiasm, it's vital to recognize the unpredictable nature of childbirth, possibly unanticipated effects, and measures for adequate pain management. This detailed analysis looks into these areas, presenting ideas to help you manage the complexity of labour with resilience and informed choices:

1. Embracing the Unpredictable:
- Despite rigorous planning, labour is generally unexpected. Labour and delivery can unfold in unanticipated ways, challenging traditional assumptions and giving the important lesson of flexibility.

2. Exploring Unexpected Outcomes:
- Childbirth, while mostly positive, can at occasion produce unforeseen effects. From alterations in birth plans to unforeseen

medical interventions, embracing these possibilities with open-mindedness is crucial.

3. Realities of Pain:
- Pain is an integral element of labour, changing in intensity and length. Understanding that pain serves a role and arming yourself with diverse pain management options will help you tackle this part.

4. Options for Pain Management:
- Childbirth offers a range of pain management solutions, from natural treatments like breathing exercises, movement, and relaxation to sophisticated methods like epidurals and medications. Educate yourself on the choices available and make informed conclusions that meet your interests.

5. Pain Management During Labor:
- Active labour frequently means rising pain. Staying flexible, applying breathing strategies, receiving massages, and utilising labour positions can bring relief and keep a sense of control.

6. Medical Interventions and Unexpected Outcomes:
- Childbirth occasionally needs medical procedures such as induced labour, episiotomy, or caesarean sections. Understanding the logic behind these acts and anticipated effects is crucial.

7. Managing Fear and Anxiety:
- Childbirth can trigger dread and anxiety, affecting the experience. Practising mindfulness, participating in relaxation techniques, and fostering a supportive culture can assist in managing emotional stress.

8. Support from Healthcare Professionals:

- Building a strong rapport with your healthcare team is crucial. Discussing hypothetical problems, remedies, and pain management techniques with them helps establish trust and open communication.

9. Birth Plans and Flexibility:
- While birth plans offer guidance, remain open to flexibility. Unexpected occurrences may demand adaptations, and embracing change can lead to a more joyful experience.

10. Empowerment Through Education:
- Knowledge helps you to make knowledgeable conclusions. Attend childbirth education sessions, study trustworthy literature, and connect with experienced parents to get suggestions.

11. Birth Support and Advocacy:
- Having a supportive birth partner, doula, or advocate can provide emotional and physical assistance, ensuring your preferences are respected.

12.   Creating   a   Supportive   Birth Environment:
- Tailor your birth environment to enhance comfort and relaxation. Dim lighting, peaceful music, and familiar scents can contribute to a tranquil mood.

13. Honouring Your Experience:
- Childbirth is a deeply personal journey. Embrace the events, sensations, and experiences that arise, regardless of how different they may be from your expectations.

14. Post-Birth Reflection:
- Reflect on your delivery experience, remembering the successes, trials, and the tremendous courage you displayed during the journey.

15. Embracing the Unpredictability of Parenthood:
- Childbirth is the prelude to the uncertain path of parenthood. By embracing the uncertainties of childbirth with resilience, you're preparing yourself for the dynamic and transforming journey ahead.

Childbirth's unpredictability is a tribute to the awe-inspiring complexity of bringing life into the world. By admitting the potential for unexpected results, examining pain management solutions, and comprehending the realities of labour, you're embracing the trip with a sense of empowerment and readiness.

Always remember that every twist and turn, every decision and choice, contributes to your unique tale as a parent. As you embark on this altering event, understand that your capacity to handle the unanticipated indicates the depth of your love and

devotion to bringing your baby into a world
teeming with possibilities.

Chapter 8

LIFE AFTER BIRTH

The journey of childbirth is a spectacular and altering experience, marking the beginning of a new chapter full of delights, challenges, and transformations.

While the attention typically centres on pregnancy and labour, it's crucial to recognize the physical and mental changes that linger after childbirth. This extensive analysis looks into the postpartum phase, giving insights on the complexities of the journey and solutions for conquering the hurdles that arise:

1. Physical Recovery:
- After childbirth, your body undergoes a process of healing and recovery. Addressing physical changes with patience and care is crucial. Be prepared for changes like vaginal

pain, perineal discomfort, and uterine contractions as your body returns to its pre-pregnancy state.

2. Hormonal Shifts:
- Hormones play a major impact on postpartum experiences. While oestrogen and progesterone levels drop, prolactin rises to support lactation. These hormonal fluctuations could contribute to mood swings, tiredness, and emotional changes.

3. Postpartum Bleeding:
- Lochia, the discharge after childbirth, is part of the body's normal healing process. Understand the different stages of postpartum bleeding and follow prescribed instructions for hygiene and care.

4. Breast Changes:
- If you're breastfeeding, your breasts will suffer changes such as engorgement, leaking, and possibly discomfort. Proper breastfeeding practices, wearing nursing

bras, and obtaining help from lactation consultants can ease these changes.

5. Caesarean Section Recovery:
- Recovering after a caesarean section comprises abdominal healing. Follow your healthcare provider's instructions for incision care, reducing pain, and gradually reintroducing physical activity.

6. Urinary and Bowel Changes:
- The pressure of childbirth and hormonal changes could contribute to pee incontinence and constipation. Pelvic floor exercises and a balanced diet can aid in treating these concerns.

7. Hair and Skin Changes:
- Hormonal swings may impact hair texture and skin concerns. Stay hydrated, use gentle skincare products, and focus on a balanced diet to ensure healthy hair and skin.

8. Fatigue and Sleep Deprivation:
- Caring for a newborn can interrupt sleep patterns and add to tiredness. Prioritise relaxation when practical, and try enlisting the support of loved ones to share childcare chores.

9. Emotional Adjustments:
- The emotional changes experienced during pregnancy can remain postpartum. The combination of hormonal shifts, sleep loss, and the demands of parenthood can contribute to mood swings, anxiety, and even postpartum depression.

10. Bonding & Attachment:
- Building a tight bond with your infant takes time. Engaging in skin-to-skin contact, exercising responsive parenting, and seeking support can build a profound attachment.

11. Body Image Concerns:
- Adjusting to your postpartum body can be tricky. Embrace self-acceptance and recognize that your body's changes represent the beautiful experience of generating a new life.

12. Relationship Dynamics:
- The arrival of a baby can alter your connection with your partner. Open communication, patience, and sharing child care chores can help preserve a healthy partnership.

13. Social Isolation:
- Adjusting to parenting can sometimes lead to feelings of isolation. Joining postpartum support groups, socialising with other parents, and seeking social connection helps ease loneliness.

14. Self-Care:
- Prioritise self-care, even in the midst of caring for a newborn. Taking occasional

pauses, engaging in things you enjoy, and getting help when needed are vital for your well-being.

15. Seeking Help:
- If you're battling with emotional shifts, exhaustion, or heavy duties, don't hesitate to seek expert help. A healthcare provider or mental health expert can offer direction and assistance.

16. Nutrition and Exercise:
- Nourishing your body with a healthy diet can promote both your physical recovery and mental well-being. Include nutrient-rich foods, stay hydrated, and consider visiting a healthcare provider before resuming exercise.

17. Managing Expectations:
- It's crucial to control your expectations throughout the postpartum time. Give yourself permission to experience a range of

emotions, challenges, and accomplishments as you navigate this new era of life.

18. Time Management:
- Balancing the demands of a newborn and your personal needs can be tough. Create a flexible regimen that allows time for self-care, bonding, and personal activities.

19. Patience and Acceptance:
- Postpartum healing is a gradual process. Patience and self-acceptance are crucial as you negotiate the changes in your body, emotions, and lifestyle.

20. Seeking Support:
- You don't have to navigate the postpartum journey alone. Lean on your partner, family, friends, and support groups for advice, encouragement, and companionship.

21. Embracing Flexibility:
- Parenthood is full of surprises, and adaptation is vital. Adapt to changes and

obstacles with an open heart, understanding that your ability to adjust contributes to your progress as a parent.

22. Self-Expression and Creativity:
- Engaging in artistic activities can be therapeutic. Whether it's journaling, drawing, or creating, expressing oneself can help process emotions and discover moments of delight.

23. Time for Intimacy:
- As a partnership, it's vital to keep emotional and physical connection. Communicate freely about your needs, seek moments of connection, and try scheduling daycare for meaningful time together.

24. Asking for Help:
- Recognize that asking for help is a show of strength, not weakness. Accept aid from friends or family members, and don't hesitate to delegate chores to lighten your load.

25. Self-Discovery and Growth:
- The postpartum phase is an adventure of self-discovery and progress. Embrace the opportunity to learn about yourself, your abilities, and the eternal love you have for your child.

26. Reflect and Celebrate:
- Take pauses to reflect on your postpartum journey and celebrate your milestones. From your baby's first smile to your own triumphs, each achievement is worth acknowledging.

27. Stay Connected with Others:
- Connect with fellow parents who are also navigating the postpartum period. Sharing experiences, providing advice, and offering support can develop a sense of camaraderie.

28. Establishing Boundaries:
- Prioritise your well-being by creating clear limits with guests, work-related expectations, and personal obligations. Protect your time for self-care and bonding with your newborn.

29. Mindful Moments:
- Incorporate mindfulness practices into your regular routine. Whether it's meditation, deep breathing, or simply savouring peaceful times, mindfulness helps enhance emotional balance.

30. Celebrating Progress:
- Reflect on your postpartum experience and acknowledge your progress. Celebrate your capacity to overcome problems, gain new skills, and adjust to your evolving position as a parent.

The postpartum time is a transforming phase that brings a blend of joys, changes, and discoveries. By treating the physical and emotional changes that persist after childbirth, you're nurturing yourself and developing a foundation of well-being for both you and your kid.

Remember that every struggle you face is an opportunity for growth, every moment of self-care is an investment in your future, and every feeling you experience is a reflection of your love and dedication as a parent. With resilience, compassion, and a desire to accept the journey, you're cultivating a life full of meaning, connection, and a meaningful bond with your lovely little one.